LEA GREEN RECIPES FOR BEGINNERS

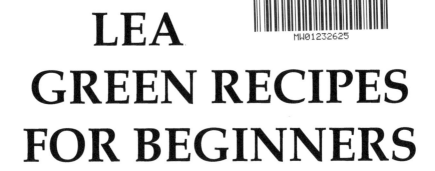
MW01232625

Very Simple Super Fast, and Tasty Recipes lo Lose Weight Easy by Using a Simple Lean and Green Cookbook

Evelyn West

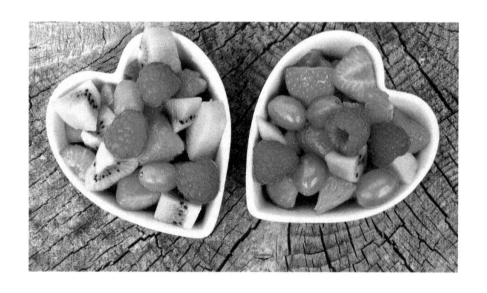

Table Of Contents

Introduction

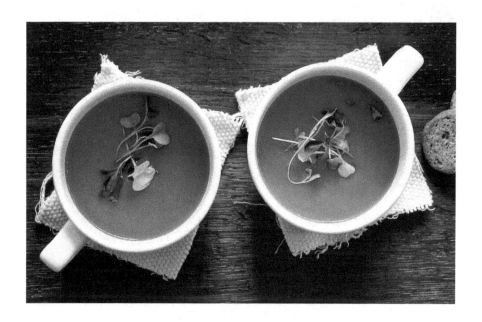

The Optavia diet focuses on making changes in your diet plan that will actually increase the metabolism of your body, while also allowing the body to obtain the adequate nutrition for building new muscle.

The basic Optavia diet is a very simple. For one month, people on the Optavia diet eat between 1000 and 1500 calorie meals.

Optavia is a diet plan that entails eating a restricted-calorie diet with specific lean protein, fat, fiber, and carbohydrates. It is linked to an app that you have to use for one month for optimum results, and if you choose to renew the app it is USD$57. The app helps you plan your meals and allows you to input your weight, activity level, goals, and food preferences to produce results that match your needs.

The diet that they provide takes into account the fact that you lose weight faster and more consistently when you are on a diet that restricts your calories. It is rare for people to consistently over-eat fat and protein; even though this may happen from time to time. However, most people under-eat healthy fats and healthy protein regularly. They also provide you with a tracker to help you monitor your protein and fat intake. The goal targets include that you should lose a specific amount of weight per week and that you should burn a specific number of calories each week. I found the idea of a goal target to be very motivating. I was also happy to note that you are not locked into a certain number of pounds per week. I believe that is not a healthy way to go about losing weight.

This diet uses lean protein and good fats as the basis for the diet. I found this to be very interesting because I had not heard of this concept before. I believe it is an excellent idea. I see protein and good fats as essential for a healthy diet. They also provide you with certain food products, like the Optavia Fix. The Optivia Fix is a package of meal bars, baked food items like bread and cookies that work with the app. Their purpose is to make it easier to follow the diet. There are also some prepackaged meals and snacks, such as lunches and dinners, that they provide. The app also allows you to alter your food plan for certain days if you want to switch things up.

One of the common issues with this diet is that it can be hard to follow due to the lack of variety, especially in the early stages. It can also be expensive, especially if you choose to get the full Optavia Diet.

What Is the Effect of The Optavia Diet on Health?

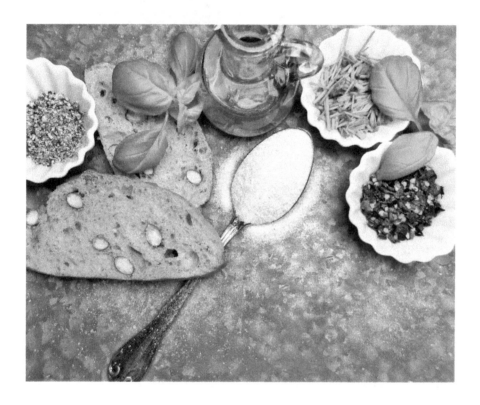

Most "supplies" contain between 100 and 110 calories each, which means you can consume around 1000 calories a day on this diet. As a result of this approach, the US News and World Report ranked it second on its list of the best diets for fast weight loss, but 32nd on its list of the best diets for healthy eating. London recognizes that there are other ways to lasting weight loss: "Eat meals and snacks that incorporate lots of products, seeds, nuts, greens, 100% whole grains, eggs, seafood, poultry, greens, low-fat dairy products. Fat, lean meat plus a little indulgence is the best way to lose weight sustainably in the long run. " So, will the Optavia diet help you lose weight?

The amount of weight you lose after following the OPTAVIA diet programs depends on factors such as your starting weight, as well as your activity and loyalty to following the plan. OPTAVIA, launched in 2017, represents the Medifast lifestyle brand and the coaching community. Previous studies have been done using Medifast products, not the new OPTAVIA products. Although the OPTAVIA products represent a new line, Medifast reported to US News that they have an identical macronutrient profile, making them interchangeable with Medifast products. Consequently, we believe that the following studies are applicable in the evaluation of this diet. Little specific research has been published on the OPTAVIA brand. The studies, like most diets, were small, with numerous dropouts. Research seems to confirm this. On the other hand, the long-term expectation is less promising

According to a 2016 study published in the journal Obesity and with partial support from Medifast, obese adults lost 8.8% of their body weight after 12 weeks with OPTAVIA style training and Medifast products, and also 12, 1% of your body weight if you were taking phentermine at the same time, which is a weight loss drug that can reduce binge eating.

However, the researchers found only one long-term study, which indicated no benefit for these 12-month plans. The researchers found that there is also an increased risk of complications, such as gallstones, on ultra-low-calorie programs.

During a small study, designed and funded by Medifast and published in 2010 in the Nutrition Journal, 90 obese adults were randomly assigned to either the low-calorie diet or the 5 & 1 plan according to government guidelines. Eventually, about half of the Medifast group and more than half of the control group withdrew.

According to a Medifast-funded study of 119 overweight or obese type 2 diabetics published in Diabetes Educator in 2008, dieters were randomly assigned to either a Medifast diabetes plan or a diet based on the recommendations of the American Association of Diabetes. After 34 weeks, the Medifast group had lost an average of 4.5 kilos, but had regained almost 1.5 kilos after 86 weeks. Over 34 weeks, those who followed the ADA-based diet lost an average of 3 pounds; they got everything back plus an extra pound in 86 weeks. By the end of the year, about 80% had given up

According to an analysis funded by Medifast and published in 2008 in the journal Eating and Weight Disorders, researchers analyzed the medical records of 324 people who were on a diet who were overweight or obese and who were also taking a prescription appetite suppressant. In 12 weeks, they lost an average of 21 pounds, in 24 weeks they weighed 26 1/2 pounds, and 27 pounds in 52 weeks.

Furthermore, for approximately 80% of them, at least 5% of the initial weight had been lost in all three evaluations. This is great if you are obese, because losing just 5-10% of your current weight can help prevent some diseases.

However, these numbers are accompanied by some asterisks. First, because they are based on people who completed or completed the 52-week program, they were more likely to lose weight. (Weight loss was still effective, but less pronounced in a cessation analysis.) Second, a review of patient data is given less importance than a study with a control group. Finally, in a survey in which researchers divided dieters into consumer groups on Medifast, that is, those who recognized that they consume at least two shakes a day at each check-in and those who are inconsistent, it is say, the rest. , weight loss was not significantly different

In a 2013 study in the International Journal of Obesity that looked at 120 men and women ages 19 to 65, half of whom were using Medifast, while the other half were limited to cutting calories, researchers found that those who on the Medifast diet lost an average of 16 1/2 pounds after 26 weeks, compared to the control group, who lost 4 kg.

Breakfast and Smoothies Recipes

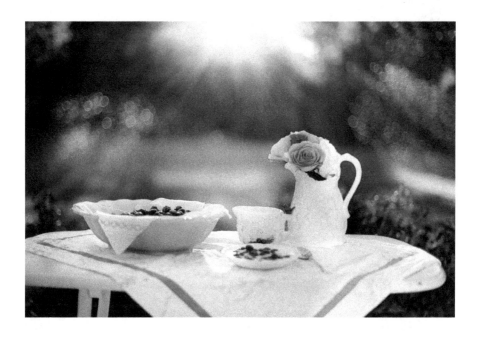

1. Chia Seed Gel with Pomegranate and Nuts

Preparation Time: 5 minutes
Cooking Time: 10 minutes
Servings: 3
Ingredients:

- 20 g hazelnuts
- 20 g walnuts
- 120 ml almond milk
- 4 tbsp chia seeds
- 4 tbsp pomegranate seeds
- 1 teaspoon agave syrup
- Some lime juices

Directions:

1. Finely chop the nuts.
2. Mix the almond milk with the chia seeds.
3. Let everything soak for 10 to 20 minutes.
4. Occasionally stir the mixture with the chia seeds.
5. Stir in the agave syrup.
6. Pour 2 tablespoons of each mixture into a dessert glass.
7. Layer the chopped nuts on top.
8. Cover the nuts with 1 tablespoon each of the chia mass.
9. Sprinkle the pomegranate seeds on top and serve everything.

Nutrition:
kcal: 248
Carbohydrates: 7 g
Protein: 1 g
Fat: 19 g

2. Lavender Blueberry Chia Seed Pudding

Preparation Time: 1 hour 10 minutes
Cooking Time: 0 minutes
Servings: 4
Ingredients:

- 100 g blueberries
- 70 g organic quark
- 50 g soy yogurt
- 30 g hazelnuts
- 200 ml almond milk
- 2 tbsp chia seeds
- 2 teaspoons agave syrup
- 2 teaspoons of lavender

Directions:

1. Bring the almond milk to a boil along with the lavender.
2. Let the mixture simmer for 10 minutes at a reduced temperature.
3. Let them cool down afterwards.
4. If the milk is cold, add the blueberries and puree everything.
5. Mix the whole thing with the chia seeds and agave syrup.
6. Let everything soak in the refrigerator for an hour.
7. Mix the yogurt and curd cheese.
8. Add both to the crowd.
9. Divide the pudding into glasses.
10. Finely chop the hazelnuts and sprinkle them on top.

Nutrition:
kcal: 252
Carbohydrates: 12 g
Protein: 1 g
Fat: 11 g

3. Yogurt with Granola and Persimmon

Preparation Time: 5 minutes
Cooking Time: 5 minutes
Servings: 1
Ingredients:

- 150g Greek style yogurt
- 20g oatmeal
- 60g fresh persimmons
- 30 ml of tap water

Directions:

1. Put the oatmeal in the pan without any fat.
2. Toast them, stirring constantly, until golden brown.
3. Then put them on a plate and let them cool down briefly.
4. Peel the persimmon and put it in a bowl with the water. Mix the whole thing into a fine puree.
5. Put the yogurt, the toasted oatmeal, and the puree in layers in a glass and serve.

Nutrition:
kcal: 286
Carbohydrates: 29 g
Protein: 1 g
Fat: 11 g

4. Smoothie Bowl with Spinach, Mango and Muesli

Preparation Time: 10 minutes
Cooking Time: 0 minutes
Servings: 1
Ingredients:

- 150g yogurt
- 30g apple
- 30g mango
- 30g low carb muesli
- 10g spinach
- 10g chia seeds

Directions:

1. Soak the spinach leaves and let them drain.
2. Peel the mango and cut it into strips.
3. Remove apple core and cut it into pieces.
4. Put everything except the mango together with the yogurt in a blender and make a fine puree out of it.
5. Put the spinach smoothie in a bowl.
6. Add the muesli, chia seeds, and mango.
7. Serve the whole thing

Nutrition:
kcal: 362
Carbohydrates: 21 g
Protein: 12 g Fat: 21 g

5. Fried Egg with Bacon

Preparation Time: 5 minutes
Cooking Time: 10 minutes
Servings: 1
Ingredients:

- 2 eggs
- 30 grams of bacon
- 2 tbsp olive oil
- salt
- pepper

Directions:

1. Heat oil in the pan and fry the bacon.
2. Reduce the heat and beat the eggs in the pan.
3. Cook the eggs and season with salt and pepper.
4. Serve the fried eggs hot with the bacon.

Nutrition:

kcal: 405

Carbohydrates: 1 g

Protein: 19 g

Fat: 38 g

6. Smoothie Bowl with Berries, Poppy Seeds, Nuts and Seeds

Preparation Time: 15 minutes
Cooking Time: 0 minutes
Servings: 2
Ingredients:

- 5 chopped almonds
- 2 chopped walnuts
- 1 apple
- ¼ banana
- 300 g yogurt
- 60 g raspberries
- 20 g blueberries
- 20 g rolled oats, roasted in a pan
- 10 g poppy seeds
- 1 teaspoon pumpkin seeds
- Agave syrup

Directions:

1. Clean the fruit and let it drain.
2. Take some berries and set them aside.
3. Place the remaining berries in a tall mixing vessel.
4. Cut the banana into slices. Put a few aside.
5. Add the rest of the banana to the berries.
6. Remove the core of the apple and cut it into quarters.
7. Cut the quarters into thin wedges and set a few aside.
8. Add the remaining wedges to the berries.
9. Add the yogurt to the fruits and mix everything into a puree.
10. Sweeten the smoothie with the agave syrup.

11. Divide it into two bowls.
12. Serve it with the remaining fruit, poppy seeds, oatmeal, nuts and seeds.

Nutrition: kcal: 284 Carbohydrates: 21 g
Protein: 11 g Fat: 19 g

7. Whole Grain Bread and Avocado

Preparation Time: 5 minutes
Cooking Time: 0 minutes
Serving: 1
Ingredients:
- 2 slices of whole meal bread
- 60 g of cottage cheese
- 1 stick of thyme
- ½ avocado
- ½ lime
- Chili flakes
- salt
- pepper

Directions:
1. Cut the avocado in half.
2. Remove the pulp and cut it into slices.
3. Pour the lime juice over it.
4. Wash the thyme and shake it dry.
5. Remove the leaves from the stem.
6. Brush the whole wheat bread with the cottage cheese.
7. Place the avocado slices on top.
8. Top with the chili flakes and thyme.
9. Add salt and pepper and serve.

Nutrition:
kcal: 490 Carbohydrates: 31 g
Protein: 19 g Fat: 21 g

8. Porridge with Walnuts

Preparation Time: 5 minutes
Cooking Time: 10 minutes
Servings: 1
Ingredients:
- 50 g raspberries
- 50 g blueberries
- 25 g of ground walnuts
- 20 g of crushed flaxseed
- 10 g of oatmeal
- 200 ml nut drink
- Agave syrup
- ½ teaspoon cinnamon
- salt

Directions:
1. Warm the nut drink in a small saucepan.
2. Add the walnuts, flaxseed, and oatmeal, stirring constantly.
3. Stir in the cinnamon and salt.
4. Simmer for 8 minutes.
5. Keep stirring everything.
6. Sweet the whole thing.
7. Put the porridge in a bowl.
8. Wash the berries and let them drain.
9. Add them to the porridge and serve everything.

Nutrition:
kcal: 378
Carbohydrates: 11 g
Protein: 18 g
Fat: 27 g

Lunch Recipes

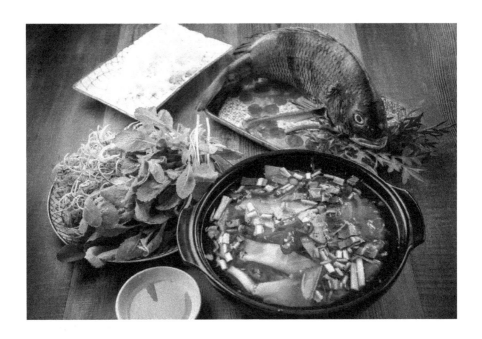

9. Crab Cakes

Preparation Time: 20 minutes
Cooking Time: 10 minutes
Servings: 2
Ingredients:
- ½ pound lump crabmeat, drained
- 2 tablespoons coconut flour
- 1 tablespoon mayonnaise
- ¼ teaspoon green Tabasco sauce
- 3 tablespoons butter
- 1 small egg, beaten
- ¾ tablespoon fresh parsley, chopped
- ½ teaspoon yellow mustard
- Salt and black pepper, to taste

Directions:
1. Mix all the ingredients in a bowl except butter.
2. Make patties from this mixture and set aside.
3. Heat butter in a skillet over medium heat and add patties.
4. Cook for about 10 minutes on each side and dish out to serve hot.
5. You can store the raw patties in the freezer for about 3 weeks for meal prepping. Place patties in a container and place parchment paper in between the patties to avoid stickiness.

Nutrition:
Calories: 153 Fat: 10.8g
Carbs: 6.7g
Protein: 6.4g
Sugar: 2.4
Sodium: 46mg

10.   Salmon Burgers

Preparation Time: 17 minutes
Cooking Time: 3 minutes
Servings: 2
Ingredients:

- 1 tablespoon sugar-free ranch dressing
- ½-ounce smoked salmon, chopped roughly
- ½ tablespoon fresh parsley, chopped
- ½ tablespoon avocado oil
- 1 small egg
- 4-ounce pink salmon, drained and bones removed
- 1/8 cup almond flour
- ¼ teaspoon Cajun seasoning

Directions:

1. Mix all the ingredients in a bowl and stir well.
2. Make patties from this mixture and set aside.
3. Heat a skillet over medium heat and add patties.
4. Cook for about 3 minutes per side and dish out to serve.
5. You can store the raw patties in the freezer for about 3 weeks for meal prepping. Place patties in a container and place parchment paper in between the patties to avoid stickiness.

Nutrition:
Calories: 59
Fat: 12.7g
Carbs: 2.4g
Protein: 6.3g
Sugar: 0.7g
Sodium: 25mg

11.   Low Carb Black Beans Chili Chicken

Preparation Time: 10 minutes
Cooking Time: 25 minutes
Servings: 10
Ingredients:

- 1-3/4 pounds of chicken breasts, cubed (boneless skinless)
- 2 sweet red peppers, chopped
- 1 onion, chopped
- 3 tablespoons of olive oil
- 1 can of chopped green chiles
- 4 cloves of garlic, minced
- 2 tablespoons of chili powder
- 2 teaspoons of ground cumin
- 1 teaspoon of ground coriander
- 2 cans of black beans, rinsed and drained
- 1 can of Italian stewed tomatoes, cut up
- 1 cup of chicken broth or beer
- 1/2 to 1 cup of water

Directions:

1. Put oil into a skillet and place over medium heat. Add in the red pepper, chicken, and onion and cook until the chicken is brown, about five minutes.
2. Add in the garlic, chiles, chili powder, coriander, and cumin and cook for an additional minute.
3. Next, add in the tomatoes, beans, half cup of water, and broth and cook until it boils. Decrease the heat, uncover the skillet and cook while stirring for fifteen minutes.
4. Serve.

Nutrition:
Calories: 236 Fat: 6g
Protein: 22g
Carbohydrates: 21g

12.   Flavorful Taco Soup

Preparation Time: 5 minutes
Cooking Time: 15
Servings: 8
Ingredients:

- 1 lb of Ground beef
- 3 tablespoons of Taco seasoning, divided
- 4 cup of Beef bone broth
- 2 14.5-oz cans of Diced tomatoes
- 3/4 cup of Ranch dressing

Directions:

1. Put the ground beef into a pot and place over medium high heat and cook until brown, about ten minutes.
2. Add in ¾ cup of broth and two tablespoons of taco seasoning. Cook until part of the liquid has evaporated.
3. Add in the diced tomatoes, rest of the broth, and rest of the taco seasoning. Stir to mix, then simmer for ten minutes.
4. Remove the pot from heat, and add in the ranch dressing. Garnish with cilantro and cheddar cheese. Serve.

Nutrition:
Calories: 309
Fat: 24g
Protein: 13g

13. Delicious Instant Pot Buffalo Chicken Soup

Preparation Time: 10 minutes
Cooking Time: 20 minutes
Servings: 6
Ingredients:

- 1 tablespoon of Olive oil
- 1/2 Onion, diced)
- 1/2 cup of Celery, diced
- 4 cloves of Garlic, minced
- 1 lb of Shredded chicken, cooked
- 4 cup of Chicken bone broth, or any chicken broth
- 3 tablespoons of Buffalo sauce
- 6 oz of Cream cheese
- 1/2 cup of Half & half

Directions:

1. Switch the instant pot to the saute function. Add in the chopped onion, oil, and celery. Cook until the onions are brown and translucent, about ten minutes.
2. Add in the garlic and cook until fragrant, about one minute. Switch off the instant pot.
3. Add in the broth, shredded chicken, and buffalo sauce. Cover the instant pot and seal. Switch the soup feature on and set time to five minutes.
4. When cooked, release pressure naturally for five minutes and then quickly.
5. Scoop out one cup of the soup liquid into a blender bowl, then add in the cheese and blend until smooth. Pour the puree into the instant pot, then add in the calf and half and stir to mix.
6. Serve.

Nutrition:
Servings: 1 cup
Calories: 270
Protein: 27g
Fat: 16g
Carbohydrates: 4g

14. Creamy Low Carb Cream of Mushroom Soup

Preparation Time: 15 minutes
Cooking Time: 15 minutes
Servings: 5
Ingredients:

- 1 tablespoons of Olive oil
- 1/2 Onion, diced
- 20 oz of Mushrooms, sliced
- 6 cloves of Garlic, minced
- 2 cup of Chicken broth
- 1 cup of Heavy cream
- 1 cup of Unsweetened almond milk
- 3/4 teaspoon of Sea salt
- 1/4 teaspoon of Black pepper

Directions:

1. Place a pot over medium heat and add in olive oil. Add in the mushrooms and onions and cook until browned, about fifteen minutes. Next, add in the garlic and cook for another one minute.
2. Add in the cream, chicken broth, sea salt, almond milk, and black pepper. Cook until boil, then simmer for fifteen minutes.
3. Puree the soup using an immersion blender until smooth. Serve.

Nutrition:
Servings: 1 cup
Calories: 229
Fat: 21g
Protein: 5g / Carbohydrates: 8g

15.   Tropical Greens Smoothie

Preparation Time: 5 Minutes
Cooking Time: 0 Minutes
Servings: 1
Ingredients:

- One banana
- 1/2 large navel orange, peeled and segmented
- 1/2 cup frozen mango chunks
- 1 cup frozen spinach
- One celery stalk, broken into pieces
- One tablespoon cashew butter or almond butter
- 1/2 tablespoon spiraling
- 1/2 tablespoon ground flaxseed
- 1/2 cup unsweetened nondairy milk
- Water, for thinning (optional)

Directions:

1. In a high-speed blender or food processor, combine the bananas, orange, mango, spinach, celery, cashew butter, spiraling (if using), flaxseed, and milk.

   2. Blend until creamy, adding more milk or water to thin the smoothie if too thick. Serve immediately — it is best served fresh.

Nutrition:
Calories: 391 Fat: 12g
Protein: 13g
Carbohydrates: 68g
Fiber: 13g

Salad Recipes

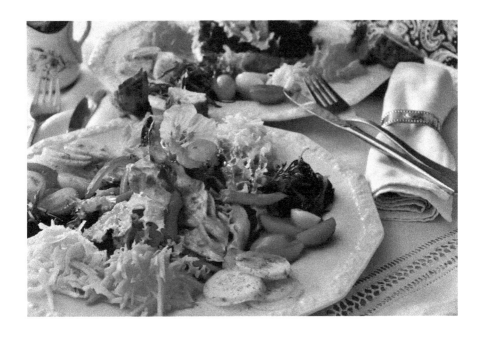

16.   Taste of Normandy Salad

Preparation Time: 25 minutes
Cooking Time: 5 minutes
Servings: 4 to 6
Ingredients:
For the walnuts:

- 2 tablespoons butter
- ¼ cup sugar or honey
- 1 cup walnut pieces
- ½ teaspoon kosher salt
- For the dressing
- 3 tablespoons extra-virgin olive oil
- 1½ tablespoons champagne vinegar
- 1½ tablespoons Dijon mustard
- ¼ teaspoon kosher salt

For the salad:

- 1 head red leaf lettuce, torn into pieces
- 3 heads endive, ends trimmed and leaves separated
- 2 apples, cored and cut into thin wedges
- 1 (8-ounce) Camembert wheel, cut into thin wedges

Directions:

1. To make the walnuts
2. In a skillet over medium-high heat, melt the butter. Stir in the sugar and cook until it dissolves. Add the walnuts and cook for about 5 minutes, stirring, until toasty. Season with salt and transfer to a plate to cool.
3. To make the dressing
4. In a large bowl, whisk the oil, vinegar, mustard, and salt until combined.
5. To make the salad

6. Add the lettuce and endive to the bowl with the dressing and toss to coat. Transfer to a serving platter.

7. Decoratively arrange the apple and Camembert wedges over the lettuce and scatter the walnuts on top. Serve immediately.

Nutrition:

Calories: 699;

Total fat: 52g;

Total carbs: 44g;

Cholesterol: 60mg;

Fiber: 17g; Protein: 23g;

Sodium: 1170mg

17.   Norwegian Niçoise Salad: Smoked Salmon, Cucumber, Egg, and Asparagus

Preparation Time: 20 minutes
Cooking Time: 5 minutes
Servings: 4
Ingredients:

- For the vinaigrette
- 3 tablespoons walnut oil
- 2 tablespoons champagne vinegar
- 1 tablespoon chopped fresh dill
- ½ teaspoon kosher salt
- ¼ teaspoon ground mustard
- Freshly ground black pepper

For the salad:

- Handful green beans, trimmed
- 1 (3- to 4-ounce) package spring greens
- 12 spears pickled asparagus
- 4 large soft-boiled eggs, halved
- 8 ounces smoked salmon, thinly sliced
- 1 cucumber, thinly sliced
- 1 lemon, quartered

Directions:

1. To make the dressing
2. In a small bowl, whisk the oil, vinegar, dill, salt, ground mustard, and a few grinds of pepper until emulsified. Set aside.
3. To make the salad
4. Start by blanching the green beans: Bring a pot of salted water to a boil. Drop in the beans. Cook or 1 to 2 minutes

until they turn bright green, then immediately drain and rinse under cold water. Set aside.

5. Divide the spring greens among 4 plates. Toss each serving with dressing to taste. Arrange 3 asparagus spears, 1 egg, 2 ounces of salmon, one-fourth of the cucumber slices, and a lemon wedge on each plate. Serve immediately.

Nutrition:

Calories: 257;

Total fat: 18g;

Total carbs: 6g;

Cholesterol: 199mg;

Fiber: 2g; Protein: 19g;

Sodium: 603mg

18.   Taste of Normandy Salad

Preparation Time: 25 minutes

Cooking Time: 5 minutes

Servings: 4 to 6

Ingredients:

For the walnuts

- 2 tablespoons butter
- 1/4 cup sugar or honey
- 1 cup walnut pieces
- 1/2 teaspoon kosher salt

For the dressing

- 3 tablespoons extra-virgin olive oil
- 11/2 tablespoons champagne vinegar
- 11/2 tablespoons Dijon mustard
- 1/4 teaspoon kosher salt

For the salad

- 1 head red leaf lettuce, shredded into pieces
- 3 heads endive, ends trimmed and leaves separated
- 2 apples, cored and divided into thin wedges
- 1 (8-ounce) Camembert wheel, cut into thin wedges

Directions:

1. To make the walnuts
2. Dissolve the butter in a skillet over medium high heat. Stir in the sugar and cook until it dissolves. Add the walnuts and cook for about 5 minutes, stirring, until toasty. Season with salt and transfer to a plate to cool.
3. To make the dressing
4. Whip the oil, vinegar, mustard, and salt in a large bowl until combined.
5. To make the salad
6. Add the lettuce and endive to the bowl with the dressing and toss to coat. Transfer to a serving platter.

7. Decoratively arrange the apple and Camembert wedges over the lettuce and scatter the walnuts on top. Serve immediately.
8. Meal Prep Tip: Prepare the walnuts in advance — in fact, double the quantities and use them throughout the week to add a healthy crunch to salads, oats, or simply to enjoy as a snack.

Nutrition: Calories: 699 Fat: 52g Carbs: 44g Protein: 23g

19.   Broccoli with Herbs and Cheese

Preparation Time: 8 minutes

Cooking Time: 17 minutes

Servings: 4

Ingredients:

- 1/3 cup grated yellow cheese
- 1 large-sized head broccoli, stemmed and cut small florets
- 2 1/2 tablespoons canola oil
- 2 teaspoons dried rosemary
- 2 teaspoons dried basil
- Salt and ground black pepper, to taste

Directions:

1. Bring a medium pan filled with a lightly salted water to a boil. Then, boil the broccoli florets for about 3 minutes.
2. Then, drain the broccoli florets well; toss them with the canola oil, rosemary, basil, salt and black pepper.
3. Set your oven to 390 degrees F; arrange the seasoned broccoli in the cooking basket; set the timer for 17 minutes. Toss the broccoli halfway through the cooking process.
4. Serve warm topped with grated cheese and enjoy!

Nutrition:

Calories: 111 Fat: 2.1g Carbs: 3.9g

Protein: 8.9g

20.   Potato Carrot Salad

Preparation Time: 15 Minutes

Cooking Time: 10 Minutes

Servings: 1

Ingredients:

Water

- One potato, sliced into cubes
- 1/2 carrots, cut into cubes
- 1/6 tablespoon milk
- 1/6 tablespoon Dijon mustard
- 1/24 cup mayonnaise
- Pepper to taste
- 1/3 teaspoons fresh thyme, chopped
- 1/6 stalk celery, chopped
- 1/6 scallions, chopped
- 1/6 slice turkey bacon, cooked crispy and crumbled

Directions:

1. Fill your pot with water.
2. Place it over medium-high heat.
3. Boil the potatoes and carrots for 10 to 12 minutes or until tender.
4. Drain and let cool.
5. In a bowl, mix the milk mustard, mayo, pepper, and thyme.
6. Stir in the potatoes, carrots, and celery.
7. Coat evenly with the sauce.
8. Cover and refrigerate for 4 hours.
9. Top with the scallions and turkey bacon bits before serving.

Nutrition:

Calories 106

Fat 5.3 g

Carbohydrates 12.6 g

Protein 2 g

21.   Marinated Veggie Salad

Preparation Time: 4 Hours and 30 Minutes
Cooking Time: 3 Minutes
Servings: 1
Ingredients:

- One zucchini, sliced
- Four tomatoes, sliced into wedges
- 1/4 cup red onion, sliced thinly
- One green bell pepper, sliced
- 2 tablespoons fresh parsley, chopped
- 2 tablespoons red-wine vinegar
- 2 tablespoons olive oil
- 1 clove garlic, minced
- 1 teaspoon dried basil
- 2 tablespoons water
- Pine nuts, toasted and chopped

Directions:

1. In a bowl, combine the zucchini, tomatoes, red onion, green bell pepper, and parsley.
2. Pour the vinegar and oil into a glass jar with a lid.
3. Add the garlic, basil, and water.
4. Seal the jar and stir well to combine.
5. Pour the dressing into the vegetable mixture.
6. Cover the bowl.
7. Marinate in the refrigerator for 4 hours.
8. Garnish with the pine nuts before serving.

Nutrition:

Calories 65

Fat 4.7 g

Carbohydrates 5.3 g

Protein 0.9 g

22.   Mediterranean Salad

Preparation Time: 20 Minutes

Cooking Time: 5 Minutes

Servings: 1

Ingredients:

- 1 teaspoon balsamic vinegar
- 1/2 tablespoon basil pesto
- 1/2 cup lettuce
- 1/8 cup broccoli florets, chopped
- 1/8 cup zucchini, chopped
- 1/8 cup tomato, chopped
- 1/8 cup yellow bell pepper, chopped
- 1/2 tablespoons feta cheese, crumbled

Directions:

1. Arrange the lettuce on a serving platter.
2. Top with the broccoli, zucchini, tomato, and bell pepper.
3. In a bowl, mix the vinegar and pesto.
4. Drizzle the dressing on top.
5. Sprinkle the feta cheese and serve.

Nutrition:

Calories 100

Fat 6 g

Carbohydrates 7 g

Protein 4 g

Snack Recipes

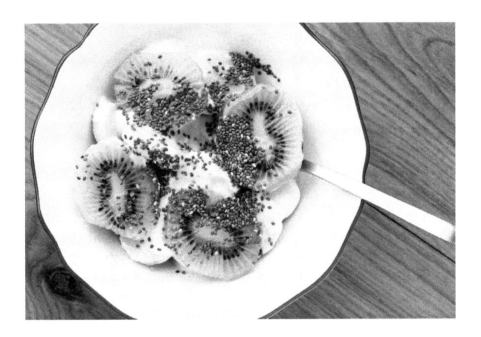

23.   Greek Baklava

Preparation Time: 20 minutes
Cooking Time: 20 minutes
Servings: 18
Ingredients:
- 1 (16 oz.) package phyllo dough
- 1 lb. chopped nuts
- 1 cup butter
- 1 teaspoon ground cinnamon
- 1 cup water
- 1 cup white sugar
- 1 teaspoon. vanilla extract
- 1/2 cup honey

Directions:
1. Preheat the oven to 175°C or 350°Fahrenheit. Spread butter on the sides and bottom of a 9-in by 13-in pan.
2. Chop the nuts then mix with cinnamon; set it aside. Unfurl the phyllo dough then halve the whole stack to fit the pan. Use a damp cloth to cover the phyllo to prevent drying as you proceed. Put two phyllo sheets in the pan then butter well. Repeat to make eight layered phyllo sheets. Scatter 2-3 tablespoons nut mixture over the sheets then place two more phyllo sheets on top, butter then sprinkle with nuts. Layer as you go. The final layer should be six to eight phyllo sheets deep.
3. Make square or diamond shapes with a sharp knife up to the bottom of pan. You can slice into four long rows for diagonal shapes. Bake until crisp and golden for 50 minutes.
4. Meanwhile, boil water and sugar until the sugar melts to make the sauce; mix in honey and vanilla. Let it simmer for 20 minutes.

5. Take the baklava out of the oven then drizzle with sauce right away; cool. Serve the baklava in cupcake papers. You can also freeze them without cover. The baklava will turn soggy when wrapped.

Nutrition:

Calories: 393 Total Carbohydrate: 37.5 g

Cholesterol: 27 mg Total Fat: 25.9 g

Protein: 6.1 g Sodium: 196 mg

24.   Glazed Bananas in Phyllo Nut Cups

Preparation Time: 30 minutes
Cooking Time: 45 minutes
Servings: 6 servings.
Ingredients:

- 3/4 cup shelled pistachios
- 1/2 cup sugar
- 1 teaspoon. ground cinnamon
- 4 sheets phyllo dough, (14 inches x 9 inches)
- 1/4 cup butter, melted

Sauce:

- 3/4 cup butter, cubed
- 3/4 cup packed brown sugar
- 3 medium firm bananas, sliced
- 1/4 teaspoon. ground cinnamon
- 3 to 4 cups vanilla ice cream

Directions:

1. Finely chop sugar and pistachios in a food processor; move to a bowl then mix in cinnamon. Slice each phyllo sheet to 6 four-inch squares, get rid of the trimmings. Pile the squares then use plastic wrap to cover.

2. Slather melted butter on each square one at a time then scatter a heaping tablespoonful of pistachio mixture. Pile 3 squares, flip each at an angle to misalign the corners. Force each stack on the sides and bottom of an oiled eight-oz. custard cup. Bake for 15-20 minutes in a 350 degrees F oven until golden; cool for 5 minutes. Move to a wire rack to completely cool.

3. Melt and boil brown sugar and butter in a saucepan to make the sauce; lower heat. Mix in cinnamon and bananas gently; heat completely. Put ice cream in the phyllo cups until full then put banana sauce on top. Serve right away.

Nutrition:
Calories: 735 Total Carbohydrate: 82 g
Cholesterol: 111 mg Total Fat: 45 g
Fiber: 3 g Protein: 7 g
Sodium: 468 mg

25.   Salmon Apple Salad Sandwich

Preparation Time: 15 minutes
Cooking Time: 10 minutes
Servings: 4
Ingredients: 4 ounces (125 g) canned pink salmon, drained and flaked

- 1 medium (180 g) red apple, cored and diced
- 1 celery stalk (about 60 g), chopped
- 1 shallot (about 40 g), finely chopped
- 1/3 cup (85 g) light mayonnaise
- 8 slices whole grain bread (about 30 g each), toasted
- 8 (15 g) Romaine lettuce leaves
- Salt and freshly ground black pepper

Directions:

1. Combine the salmon, apple, celery, shallot, and mayonnaise in a mixing bowl. Season with salt and pepper.
2. Place 1 slices bread on a plate, top with lettuce and salmon salad, and then covers with another slice of bread. Repeat procedure for the remaining ingredients.
3. Serve and enjoy.

Nutrition: Calories: 315 Fat - 11.3 g

Carbohydrates - 40.4 g Protein - 15.1 g

Sodium - 469 mg

26. Smoked Salmon and Cheese on Rye Bread

Preparation Time: 15 minutes
Cooking Time: 10 minutes
Servings: 4
Ingredients:
- 8 ounces (250 g) smoked salmon, thinly sliced
- 1/3 cup (85 g) mayonnaise
- 2 tablespoons (30 ml) lemon juice
- 1 tablespoon (15 g) Dijon mustard
- 1 teaspoon (3 g) garlic, minced
- 4 slices cheddar cheese (about 2 oz. or 30 g each)
- 8 slices rye bread (about 2 oz. or 30 g each)
- 8 (15 g) Romaine lettuce leaves
- Salt and freshly ground black pepper

Directions:
1. Mix together the mayonnaise, lemon juice, mustard, and garlic in a small bowl. Flavor with salt and pepper and set aside.
2. Spread dressing on 4 bread slices. Top with lettuce, salmon, and cheese. Cover with remaining rye bread slices.
3. Serve and enjoy.

Nutrition:
Calories: 365 Fat: 16.6 g
Carbohydrates: 31.6 g
Protein: 18.8 g
Sodium: 951 mg

27.   Pan-Fried Trout

Preparation Time: 15 minutes
Cooking Time: 10 minutes
Servings: 4
Ingredients:

- 1 ¼ pounds trout fillets
- 1/3 cup white, or yellow, cornmeal
- ¼ teaspoon anise seeds
- ¼ teaspoon black pepper
- ½ cup minced cilantro, or parsley
- Vegetable cooking spray
- Lemon wedges

Directions:

1. Coat fish with combined cornmeal, spices, and cilantro, pressing it gently into fish. Spray large skillet with cooking spray; heat over medium heat until hot.
2. Add fish and cook until fish is tender and flakes with fork, about 5 minutes on each side. Serve with lemon wedges.

Nutrition:

Calories: 207
Total Carbohydrate: 19 g
Cholesterol: 27 mg
Total Fat: 16 g
Fiber: 4 g
Protein: 18g

28.   Greek Tuna Salad Bites

Preparation Time: 5 Minutes
Cooking Time: 10 Minutes
Servings: 6
Ingredients:
- Cucumbers (2 medium)
- White tuna (2 - 6 oz. cans.)
- Lemon juice (half of 1 lemon)
- Red bell pepper (.5 cup)
- Sweet/red onion (.25 cup)
- Black olives (.25 cup)
- Garlic (2 tablespoon.)
- Olive oil (2 tablespoon.)
- Fresh parsley (2 tablespoon.)
- Dried oregano - salt & pepper (as desired)

Directions:
1. Drain and flake the tuna. Juice the lemon. Dice/chop the onions, olives, pepper, parsley, and garlic up Slice each of the cucumbers into thick rounds (skin off or on).
2. In a mixing container, combine the rest of the fixings.
3. Place a heaping spoonful of salad onto the rounds and enjoy for your next party or just a snack.

Nutrition:
Calories: 400
Fats: 22 g
Carbs: 26 g
Fiber Content: 8 g
Protein: 30 g

29. Spinach Artichoke-stuffed Chicken Breasts

Preparation Time: 15 Minutes
Cooking Time: 15 Minutes
Servings: 6
Ingredients:

- ¼ cup Greek yogurt
- ¼ cup spinach, thawed & drained
- ½ cup artichoke hearts, thinly sliced
- ½ cup mozzarella cheese, shredded
- 1 ½ lb. chicken breasts
- 2 tablespoons. olive oil
- 4 ozs. cream cheese
- Sea salt & pepper, to taste

Directions:

1. Pound the chicken breasts to a thickness of about one inch. Using a sharp knife, slice a "pocket" into the side of each. This is where you will put the filling.
2. Sprinkle the breasts with salt and pepper and set aside.
3. In a medium bowl, combine cream cheese, yogurt, mozzarella, spinach, artichoke, salt, and pepper and mix thoroughly. A hand mixer may be the easiest way to combine all the ingredients thoroughly.
4. Spoon the mixture into the pockets of each breast and set aside while you heat a large skillet over medium heat and warm the oil in it. If you have an extra filling you can't fit into the breasts, set it aside until just before your chicken is done cooking.
5. Cook each breast for about eight minutes per side, then pull off the heat when it reaches an internal temperature of about 165° Fahrenheit.

6. Just before you pull the chicken out of the pan, heat the remaining filling to warm it through and to rid it of any cross-contamination from the chicken. Once hot, top the chicken breasts with it.

7. Serve!

Nutrition:

- Calories: 238 Cal
- Fat: 22 g Carbs: 5 g

Protein: 17 g Fiber: 4 g

Dinner Recipes

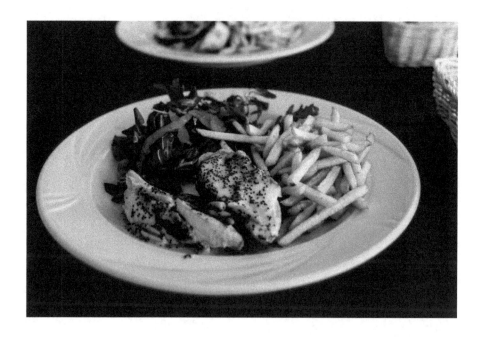

30. Sriracha Tuna Kabobs

Preparation Time: 4 minutes
Cooking Time: 9 minutes
Servings: 4
Ingredients:
- 4 T Huy Fong chili garlic sauce
- 1 T sesame oil infused with garlic
- 1 T ginger, fresh, grated
- 1 T garlic, minced
- 1 red onion, cut into quarters and separated by petals
- 2 cups bell peppers, red, green, yellow
- 1 can whole water chestnuts, cut in half
- ½ pound fresh mushrooms, halved
- 32 oz. boneless tuna, chunks or steaks
- 1 Splenda packet
- 2 zucchini, sliced 1 inch thick, keep skins on

Directions:
1. Layer the tuna and the vegetable pieces evenly onto 8 skewers.
2. Combine the spices and the oil and chili sauce, add the Splenda
3. Quickly blend, either in blender or by quickly whipping.
4. Brush onto the kabob pieces, make sure every piece is coated
5. Grill 4 minutes on each side, check to ensure the tuna is cooked to taste.
6. Serving size is two skewers.

Nutrition:
Calories: 467 Total Fat: 18g
Protein: 56g Total Carbs: 21g
Dietary Fiber: 3.5g Sugar: 6g / Sodium: 433mg

31.   Steak Salad with Asian Spice

Preparation Time: 4 minutes
Cooking Time: 4 minutes
Servings: 2
Ingredients:

- 2 T sriracha sauce
- 1 T garlic, minced
- 1 T ginger, fresh, grated
- 1 bell pepper, yellow, cut in thin strips
- 1 bell pepper, red, cut in thin strips
- 1 T sesame oil, garlic
- 1 Splenda packet
- ½ teaspoon curry powder
- ½ teaspoon rice wine vinegar
- 8 oz. of beef sirloin, cut into strips
- 2 cups baby spinach, stemmed
- ½ head butter lettuce, torn or chopped into bite-sized pieces

Directions:

1. Place the garlic, sriracha sauce, 1 teaspoon sesame oil, rice wine vinegar, and Splenda into a bowl and combine well.
2. Pour half of this mix into a zip-lock bag. Add the steak to marinade while you are preparing the salad.
3. Assemble the brightly colored salad by layering in two bowls.
4. Place the baby spinach into the bottom of the bowl.
5. Place the butter lettuce next.
6. Mix the two peppers and place on top.
7. Remove the steak from the marinade and discard the liquid and bag.
8. Heat the sesame oil and quickly stir fry the steak until desired doneness, it should take about 3 minutes.

9. Place the steak on top of the salad.

10.   Drizzle with the remaining dressing (other half of marinade mix).

11.   Sprinkle sriracha sauce across the salad.

Nutrition:

Calories: 350

Total Fat: 23g

Protein: 28g

Total Carbs: 7g

Dietary Fiber: 3.5

Sugar: 0

Sodium: 267mg

32.   Tilapia and Broccoli

Preparation Time: 4 minutes
Cooking Time: 14 minutes
Servings: 1
Ingredients:
- 6 oz. tilapia, frozen is fine
- 1 T butter
- 1 T garlic, minced or finely chopped
- 1 teaspoon of lemon pepper seasoning
- 1 cup broccoli florets, fresh or frozen, but fresh will be crisper

Directions:
1. Set the pre-warmed oven for 350 degrees.
2. Place the fish in an aluminum foil packet.
3. Arrange the broccoli around the fish to make an attractive arrangement.
4. Sprinkle the lemon pepper on the fish.
5. Close the packet and seal, bake for 14 minutes.
6. Combine the garlic and butter. Set aside.
7. Remove the packet from the oven and transfer ingredients to a plate.
8. Place the butter on the fish and broccoli.

Nutrition:
Calories: 362 Total Fat: 25g
Protein: 29g Total Carbs: 3.5g
Dietary Fiber: 3g Sugar: 0g
Sodium: 0mg

33. Brown Basmati Rice Pilaf

Preparation Time: 10 minutes
Cooking Time: 3 minutes
Servings: 2
Ingredients:

- ½ tablespoon vegan butter
- ½ cup mushrooms, chopped
- ½ cup brown basmati rice
- 2-3 tablespoons water
- 1/8 teaspoon dried thyme
- Ground pepper to taste
- ½ tablespoon olive oil
- ¼ cup green onion, chopped
- 1 cup vegetable broth
- ¼ teaspoon salt
- ¼ cup chopped, toasted pecans

Directions:

1. Place a saucepan over medium-low heat. Add butter and oil.
2. When it melts, add mushrooms and cook until slightly tender.
3. Stir in the green onion and brown rice. Cook for 3 minutes. Stir constantly.
4. Stir in the broth, water, salt, and thyme.
5. When it begins to boil, lower the heat and cover with a lid. Simmer until rice is cooked. Add more water or broth if required.
6. Stir in the pecans and pepper.
7. Serve.

Nutrition:
Calories 189 Fats 11 g / Carbohydrates 19 g Proteins 4 g

34.   Walnut and Date Porridge

Preparation Time: 10 minutes

Cooking Time: 0 minutes

Servings: 1

Ingredients:

- Strawberries, ½ cup (hulled)
- Milk or dairy-free alternative, 200 ml
- Buckwheat flakes, ½ cup
- Medjool date, 1 (chopped)
- Walnut butter, 1 teaspoon, or chopped walnut halves

Directions:

1. Place the date and the milk in a pan, heat gently before adding the buckwheat flakes. Then cook until the porridge gets to your desired consistency.
2. Add the walnuts, stir, then top with the strawberries.
3. Serve.

Nutrition:

Calories: 254 Protein: 65 g

Fat: 4 g

Vitamin B

35. Vietnamese Turmeric Fish with Mango and Herbs Sauce

Preparation Time: 15 minutes

Cooking Time: 30 minutes

Servings: 4

Ingredients:

For the Fish:

- Coconut oil to fry the fish, 2 tablespoons
- Fresh codfish, skinless and boneless, 1 ¼ lbs. (cut into 2-inch piece wide)
- Pinch of sea salt, to taste

Fish Marinade:

- Chinese cooking wine, 1 tablespoon
- Turmeric powder, 1 tablespoon
- Sea salt, 1 teaspoon
- Olive oil, 2 tablespoons
- Minced ginger, 2 teaspoons

Mango Dipping Sauce:

- Juice of ½ lime
- Medium-sized ripe mango, 1
- Rice vinegar, 2 tablespoons
- Dry red chili pepper, 1 teaspoon (stir in before serving)
- Garlic clove, 1
- Infused scallion and dill oil
- Fresh dill, 2 cups
- Scallions, 2 cups (slice into long thin shape)
- A pinch of sea salt, to taste.

Toppings

- Nuts (pine or cashew nuts)
- Lime juice (as much as you like)
- Fresh cilantro (as much as you like)

Directions:

1. Add all the ingredients under "Mango Dipping Sauce" into your food processor. Blend until you get your preferred consistency.

2. Add two tablespoons of coconut oil in a large non-stick frying pan and heat over high heat. Once hot, add the pre-marinated fish. Add the slices of the fish into the pan individually. Divide into batches for easy frying, if necessary.

3. Once you hear a loud sizzle, reduce the heat to medium-high.

4. Do not move or turn the fish until it turns golden brown on one side; then turn it to the other side to fry, about 5 minutes on each side. Add more coconut oil to the pan if needed. Season with the sea salt.

5. Transfer the fish to a large plate. You will have some oil left in the frypan, which you will use to make your scallion and dill infused oil.

6. Using the remaining oil in the frypan, set to medium-high heat, add 2 cups of dill, and 2 cups of scallions.

7. Put off the heat after you have added the dill and scallions. Toss them gently for about 15 seconds, until the dill and scallions have wilted. Add a dash of sea salt to season.

8. Pour the dill, scallion, and infused oil over the fish. Serve with mango dipping sauce, nuts, lime, and fresh cilantro.

Nutrition:
Calories: 234 Fat: 23 g
Protein: 76 g
Sugar: 5 g

36. Chicken and Kale Curry

Preparation Time: 20 min
Cooking Time: 1 hour
Servings: 3
Ingredients:

- Boiling water, 250 ml
- Skinless and boneless chicken thighs, 7 oz.
- Ground turmeric, 2 tablespoons
- Olive oil, 1 tablespoon
- Red onions, 1 (diced)
- Bird's eye chili, 1 (finely chopped)
- Freshly chopped ginger, ½ tablespoon
- Curry powder, ½ tablespoon
- Garlic, 1 ½ cloves (crushed)
- Cardamom pods, 1
- Tinned coconut milk, light, 100 ml
- Chicken stock, 2 cups
- Tinned chopped tomatoes, 1 cup

Direction:

1. Place the chicken thighs in a non-metallic bowl, add one tablespoon of turmeric and one teaspoon of olive oil. Mix together and keep aside to marinate for approx. 30 minutes.
2. Fry the chicken thighs over medium heat for about 5 minutes until well cooked and brown on all sides. Remove from the pan and set aside.
3. Add the remaining oil into a frypan on medium heat. Then add the onion, ginger, garlic, and chili. Fry for about 10 minutes until soft.

4. Add one tablespoon of the turmeric and half a tablespoon of curry powder to the pan and cook for another 2 minutes.
5. Then add the cardamom pods, coconut milk, tomatoes, and chicken stock. Allow simmering for thirty minutes.
6. Add the chicken once the sauce has reduced a little into the pan, followed by the kale. Cook until the kale is tender and the chicken is warm enough.
7. Serve with buckwheat.
8. Garnish with the chopped coriander.

Nutrition:

Calories: 313 g

Protein: 13 g

Fat: 6 g

Carbohydrate: 23 g

Side Dish Recipes

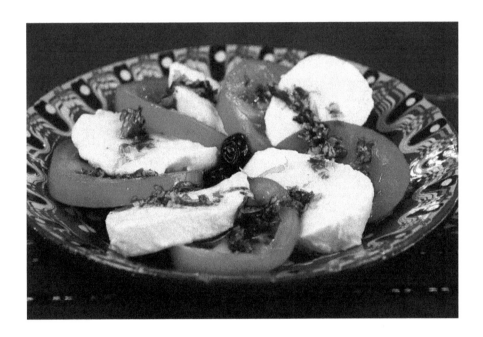

37.   Onion Green Beans

Preparation Time: 10 minutes
Cooking Time: 12 minutes
Servings: 2
Ingredients:
- 11 oz. green beans
    - 1 tablespoon onion powder
    - 1 tablespoon olive oil
    - ½ teaspoon salt
    - ¼ teaspoon chili flakes

Directions:
1. Wash the green beans carefully and place them in the bowl.
2. Sprinkle the green beans with the onion powder, salt, chili flakes, and olive oil.
3. Shake the green beans carefully.
4. Preheat the air fryer to 400 F.
5. Put the green beans in the air fryer and cook for 8 minutes.
6. After this, shake the green beans and cook them for 4 minutes more at 400 F.
7. When the time is over – shake the green beans.
8. Serve the side dish and enjoy!

Nutrition: Calories: 1205 Fat: 7.2g Fiber: 5.5g Carbs: 13.9g Protein: 3.2g

38. Mozzarella Radish Salad

Preparation Time: 10 minutes
Cooking Time: 20 minutes
Servings: 2
Ingredients:
- 8 oz. radish
    - 4 oz. Mozzarella
    - 1 teaspoon balsamic vinegar
    - ½ teaspoon salt
    - 1 tablespoon olive oil
    - 1 teaspoon dried oregano

Directions:
1. Wash the radish carefully and cut it into the halves.
2. Preheat the air fryer to 360 F.
3. Put the radish halves in the air fryer basket.
4. Sprinkle the radish with the salt and olive oil.
5. Cook the radish for 20 minutes.
6. Shake the radish after 10 minutes of cooking.
7. When the time is over – transfer the radish to the serving plate.
8. Chop Mozzarella roughly.
9. Sprinkle the radish with Mozzarella, balsamic vinegar, and dried oregano.
10. Stir it gently with the help of 2 forks.
11. Serve it immediately.

Nutrition: Calories: 241 Fat: 17.2g Fiber: 2.1g Carbs: 6.4g Protein: 16.9g

39. Cremini Mushroom Satay

Preparation Time: 10 minutes
Cooking Time: 6 minutes
Servings: 2
Ingredients:

- 7 oz. cremini mushrooms
    - 2 tablespoon coconut milk
    - 1 tablespoon butter
    - 1 teaspoon chili flakes
    - ½ teaspoon balsamic vinegar
    - ½ teaspoon curry powder
    - ½ teaspoon white pepper

Directions:

1. Wash the mushrooms carefully.
2. Then sprinkle the mushrooms with the chili flakes, curry powder, and white pepper.
3. Preheat the air fryer to 400 F.
4. Toss the butter in the air fryer basket and melt it.
5. Put the mushrooms in the air fryer and cook for 2 minutes.
6. Shake the mushrooms well and sprinkle with the coconut milk and balsamic vinegar.
7. Cook the mushrooms for 4 minutes more at 400 F.
8. Then skewer the mushrooms on the wooden sticks and serve.
9. Enjoy!

Nutrition: Calories 116 Fat: 9.5g Fiber: 1.3g Carbs: 5.6g Protein: 3g

40.   Eggplant Ratatouille

Preparation Time: 15 minutes
Cooking Time: 15 minutes
Servings: 2
Ingredients:
- 1 eggplant
  - 1 sweet yellow pepper
  - 3 cherry tomatoes
  - 1/3 white onion, chopped
  - ½ teaspoon garlic clove, sliced
  - 1 teaspoon olive oil
  - ½ teaspoon ground black pepper
  - ½ teaspoon Italian seasoning

Directions:
1. Preheat the air fryer to 360 F.
2. Peel the eggplants and chop them.
3. Put the chopped eggplants in the air fryer basket.
4. Chop the cherry tomatoes and add them to the air fryer basket.
5. Then add chopped onion, sliced garlic clove, olive oil, ground black pepper, and Italian seasoning.
6. Chop the sweet yellow pepper roughly and add it to the air fryer basket.
7. Shake the vegetables gently and cook for 15 minutes.
8. Stir the meal after 8 minutes of cooking.
9. Transfer the cooked ratatouille in the serving plates.
10. Enjoy!

Nutrition: Calories: 149 Fat: 3.7g Fiber: 11.7g Carbs: 28.9g
Protein: 5.1g

41.   Cheddar Portobello Mushrooms

Preparation Time: 15 minutes

Cooking Time: 6 minutes

Servings: 2

Ingredients:

- 2 Portobello mushroom hats
    - 2 slices Cheddar cheese
    - ¼ cup panko breadcrumbs
    - ½ teaspoon salt
    - ½ teaspoon ground black pepper
    - 1 egg
    - 1 teaspoon oatmeal
    - 2 oz. bacon, chopped cooked

Directions:

1. Crack the egg into the bowl and whisk it.
2. Combine the ground black pepper, oatmeal, salt, and breadcrumbs in the separate bowl.
3. Dip the mushroom hats in the whisked egg.
4. After this, coat the mushroom hats in the breadcrumb mixture.
5. Preheat the air fryer to 400 F.
6. Place the mushrooms in the air fryer basket tray and cook for 3 minutes.
7. After this, put the chopped bacon and sliced cheese over the mushroom hats and cook the meal for 3 minutes.
8. When the meal is cooked – let it chill

9. gently.

10. Enjoy!

Nutrition: Calories: 376 Fat: 24.1g Fiber: 1.8g Carbs: 14.6g Protein: 25.2g

42.   Salty Edamame

Preparation Time: 15 minutes

Cooking Time: 6 minutes

Servings: 2

Ingredients:

- 1 cup of edamame, inside a shell
- The salt, for taste

Directions:

1. Over a medium-low heat, place a large saucepan. Add 2 quarts of edamame and water. Cover and simmer for about 5-8 minutes, until tender.
2. Drain and add salt to sprinkle.

Nutrition: Calories: 376 Fat: 24.1g Fiber: 1.8g Carbs: 14.6g Protein: 25.2g

43. Parsley Zucchini and Radishes

Preparation time: 5 minutes
Cooking time: 15 minutes
Servings: 4
Ingredients

- 1 pound zucchinis, cubed
- 1 cup radishes, halved
- 1 tablespoon olive oil
- 1 tablespoon balsamic vinegar
- 2 tomatoes, cubed
- 3 tablespoons parsley, chopped
- Salt and black pepper to the taste

Directions

1. In a pan that fits your air fryer, mix the zucchinis with the radishes, oil and the other ingredients, toss, introduce in the fryer and cook at 350 degrees F for 15 minutes.
2. Divide between plates and serve as a side dish.
   Nutrition: Calories 170, Fat 6, Fiber 2, Carbs 5, Protein 6

Dessert Recipes

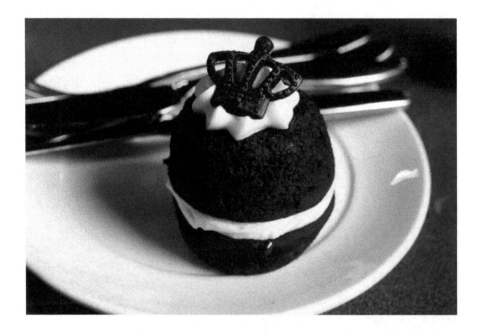

44. Chocolate Popsicle

Preparation Time: 20 minutes

Cooking Time: 10 minutes

Servings: 6

Ingredients:

- 4 oz unsweetened chocolate, chopped
- 6 drops liquid stevia
- 1 1/2 cups heavy cream

Directions:

1. Add heavy cream into the microwave-safe bowl and microwave until just begins the boiling.
2. Add chocolate into the heavy cream and set aside for 5 minutes.
3. Add liquid stevia into the heavy cream mixture and stir until chocolate is melted.
4. Pour mixture into the Popsicle molds and place in freezer for 4 hours or until set.
5. Serve and enjoy.

Nutrition: Calories: 198 Fat: 21 g Carbs: 6 g Sugar: 0.2 g Protein: 3 g Cholesterol: 41 mg

45. Raspberry Ice Cream

Preparation Time: 10 minutes

Cooking Time: 0 minutes

Servings: 2

Ingredients:

- 1 cup frozen raspberries
  - 1/2 cup heavy cream
  - 1/8 tsp stevia powder

Directions:

1. Blend all the listed ingredients in a blender until smooth.
2. Serve immediately and enjoy.

Nutrition: Calories: 144 Fat: 11 g Carbs: 10 g Sugar: 4 g Protein: 2 g Cholesterol: 41 mg

46.   Chocolate Frosty

Preparation Time: 20 minutes

Cooking Time: 0 minutes

Servings: 4

Ingredients:

- 2 tbsp unsweetened cocoa powder
  - 1 cup heavy whipping cream
  - 1 tbsp almond butter
  - 5 drops liquid stevia
  - 1 tsp vanilla

Directions:

1. Add cream into the medium bowl and beat using the hand mixer for 5 minutes.
2. Add remaining ingredients and blend until thick cream form.
3. Pour in serving bowls and place them in the freezer for 30 minutes.
4. Serve and enjoy.

Nutrition: Calories: 137 Fat: 13 g Carbs: 3 g Sugar: 0.5 g Protein: 2 g Cholesterol: 41 mg

47. Chocolate Almond Butter Brownie

Preparation Time: 10 minutes

Cooking Time: 16 minutes

Servings: 4

Ingredients:

- 1 cup bananas, overripe
  - 1/2 cup almond butter, melted
  - 1 scoop protein powder
  - 2 tbsp unsweetened cocoa powder

Directions:

1. Preheat the air fryer to 325 F. Grease air fryer baking pan and set aside.
2. Blend all ingredients in a blender until smooth.
3. Pour batter into the prepared pan and place in the air fryer basket and cook for 16 minutes.
4. Serve and enjoy.

Nutrition: Calories: 82 Fat: 2 g Carbs: 11 g Sugar: 5 g Protein: 7 g Cholesterol: 16 mg

48.   Peanut Butter Fudge

Preparation Time: 10 minutes

Cooking Time: 10 minutes

Servings: 20

Ingredients:

- 1/4 cup almonds, toasted and chopped
  - 12 oz smooth peanut butter
  - 15 drops liquid stevia
  - 3 tbsp coconut oil
  - 4 tbsp coconut cream
  - Pinch of salt

Directions:

1. Line baking tray with parchment paper.
2. Melt coconut oil in a pan over low heat. Add peanut butter, coconut cream, stevia, and salt in a saucepan. Stir well.
3. Pour fudge mixture into the prepared baking tray and sprinkle chopped almonds on top.
4. Place the tray in the refrigerator for 1 hour or until set.
5. Slice and serve.

Nutrition: Calories: 131 Fat: 12 g Carbs: 4 g Sugar: 2 g Protein: 5 g Cholesterol: 0 mg

49.   Almond Butter Fudge

Preparation Time: 10 minutes

Cooking Time: 10 minutes

Servings: 18

Ingredients:

- 3/4 cup creamy almond butter
    - 1 1/2 cups unsweetened chocolate chips

Directions:

1. Line 8*4-inch pan with parchment paper and set aside.

2.   Add chocolate chips and almond butter into the double boiler and cook over medium heat until the chocolate-butter mixture is melted. Stir well. Place mixture into the prepared pan and place in the freezer until set.

3. Slice and serve.

Nutrition: Calories: 197 Fat: 16 g Carbs: 7 g Sugar: 1 g Protein: 4 g Cholesterol: 0 mg

50.   Bounty Bars

Preparation Time: 20 minutes
Cooking Time: 0 minutes
Servings: 12
Ingredients:

- 1 cup coconut cream
- 3 cups shredded unsweetened coconut
- 1/4 cup extra virgin coconut oil
- 1/2 teaspoon vanilla powder
- 1/4 cup powdered erythritol
- 1 1/2 oz. cocoa butter
- 5 oz. dark chocolate

Directions:

1.   Heat the oven at 350 °F and toast the coconut in it for 5-6 minutes. Remove from the oven once toasted and set aside to cool.

2.   Take a bowl of medium size and add coconut oil, coconut cream, vanilla, erythritol, and toasted coconut. Mix the ingredients well to prepare a smooth mixture.

3.   Make 12 bars of equal size with the help of your hands from the prepared mixture and adjust in the tray lined with parchment paper.

4.   Place the tray in the fridge for around one hour and, in the meantime, put the cocoa butter and dark chocolate in a glass bowl.

5.   Heat a cup of water in a saucepan over medium heat and place the bowl over it to melt the cocoa butter and the dark chocolate.

6.   Remove from the heat once melted properly, mix well until blended and set aside to cool.

7.   Take the coconut bars and coat them with dark chocolate mixture one by one using a wooden stick. Adjust on the tray lined with parchment paper and drizzle the remaining mixture over them.

8.   Refrigerate for around one hour before you serve the delicious bounty bars.

Nutrition:

Calories: 230 Fat: 25 g

Carbohydrates: 5 g Protein: 32 g

Conclusion

Optavia is a weight management program that has been approved by the FDA. It is an independent initiative taken by the American Medical Association (AMA). It is a scientifically researched and proven diet program, which has been tested and found to be 100% successful . Some great benefits of Optavia over some other diet programs are:

A person can lose up to 3 pounds in the initial week of the program and continue to lose weight at a steady pace. If these 3 lbs aren't lost within 1 week, it is advisable to consult a physician .

The Optavia diet plan is Low in protein and Low in fat. and has been found to protect a person from obesity. Optavia diet does not require major lifestyle changes.

The Optavia diet is a series of three plans, two of which concentrate on weight reduction and better at managing weight. The program's foods are lower in calories and carbs and higher in protein to promote weight reduction. Each strategy demands that you consume at least half of your food in the form of Optavia pre-packaged food. Since the menu calls for eating carbs, protein, and healthy fat to be eaten, it is a reasonably healthy diet for healthy food. As far as weight reduction goes, experts agree that Optavia can benefit because its diet is low in calories, for the positive. Still, it's unlikely to change your eating habits significantly. You're likely to regain weight once you quit your diet.

Hence optavia diet has proven to be extremely helpful in controlling and maintaining weight. Still, when optavia lean & green food merges with air frying, it can make this diet much easier for people to follow. Air frying food cuts the cooking time in half and makes the food more nutritious.

The Optavia Weight Loss Plan promotes weight loss through low calorie prepackaged meals; Homemade food with easy carbohydrates and personalized coaching.The Optavia diet advances weight reduction using low calorie prepackaged foods, low carb natively constructed suppers, and customized instructing.

However, the diet is costly, repetitive, and doesn't accommodate all nutritional wishes. what's extra, Extended calorie limit may also result in nutrient deficiencies and different potential health issues.

Be that as it may, the eating routine is costly, monotonous, and doesn't suit every dietary need. Additionally, expanded calorie limitation may bring about supplement insufficiencies and other potential health concerns.

Simultaneously, as this system promotes quick-time period weight and Fat's loss, similarly research is wanted to assess whether it encourages the everlasting way of life adjustments needed for long-time period achievement.

I hope you have learned something

In a nutshell, the Optavia Diet is meant to be followed for short term, and is mainly designed to help people lose weight.

CPSIA information can be obtained
at www.ICGtesting.com
Printed in the USA
LVHW011126090621
689684LV00011B/1335